Kettlebell Workouts

One Kettlebell 100 Exercises – The Superior Soviet Approach To Absolute Fitness; Kettlebell Workouts And Kettlebell Training

Kettlebell Workouts Content

Contents

The Soviet Secret

10 years ago few people outside of the Soviet Union knew what a kettlebell was. Today it has morphed into the 'in' piece of equipment for fat loss and functional fitness. But make no mistake – kettlebells are no passing fad.

They've been around for well over a century and their time in the lime-light is well over-due. Simply put, they are one of the most time efficient ways to achieve functional whole-body fitness, while developing explosive strength and power. They're also a great way to burn through the calories and achieve peak aerobic fitness.

Here's what Kettlebells can do for you . . .

- **Improve explosive power and maximal strength**
- **Develop functional muscle mass**
- **Enhance muscular endurance**
- **Burn up to 20.2 calories per minute**
- **Promote coordination among all the muscles of the body**
- **Blast the often neglected but vital muscles of the posterior kinetic chain (the muscles you don't see in the mirror)**
- **A superior and targeted way to correct lower back issues**
- **Versatility – one kettlebell, over 100 exercises –enough said!**

In this book you will learn exactly how to use kettlebells to forge your new body. We'll show you how to handle them, how to use them in your workouts and how to build programs around them for fat loss, muscle mass and cardio fitness. It's time to start putting those weird bowling balls with handles to use!

I. Kettlebell Foundation

They may not look like much, but kettlebells are an all in one gym. As you've probably noticed, kettlebells have a unique design that sets them apart from other training apparatus out there. A kettlebell is a cast iron weight that looks very much like a cannon ball, but with a handle attached. The thing that makes this equipment super effective is the design of the handle, which allows for the center of mass of the kettlebell to extend beyond your hand. This makes the kettlebell an ideal piece of equipment for such ballistic movements as swings. Ballistic movements are a great choice because they integrate cardio, strength and flexibility training all in one awesome movement.

Ballistic movements also allow you to develop functional fitness that copies activities that we perform in the real world, such as shoveling snow.

There are two prime functions of kettlebell training:

(1) Developing functional fitness
(2) Training specifically for kettlebell competition

In this book we will focus exclusively on functional fitness movements that will rid your body of fat while building muscle, leaning you up and boosting your fitness.

Getting To Know Your Kettlebell

Kettlebells can be either fixed load or adjustable. Obviously, fixed load kettlebells are quicker and easier to use, as there is no having to change resistances between movements.

The kettlebell handle is the part of the equipment that you will most frequently come in contact with. Kettlebell handles may vary from very smooth to very rough. You want one that is neither too smooth nor too rough, but will allow for a firm grip when your hands get sweaty.

The unique shape of the kettlebell makes it a superior choice for many exercises. The shape of the weight and the distance between the handle and the ball allow for swinging and catch and release movements. It also allows the weight to sit directly against the arm, providing for greater leverage. Providing for neutral alignment of the hand and arm also allows for greater endurance of the arm muscles throughout the exercise.

The kettlebell sets in your gym will typically range from 8kg (18 pounds) to 48kg (106 pounds). The average man should start with a 16 kg (35 pound) bell, while most women begin training with an 8kg (18 pound) bell.

Clothing Considerations

Try to avoid wearing loose fitting clothing that is liable to get caught up in the kettlebell during such movements as swings. You should also stay away from slick logos and designs on your clothing that are going to make you sweat a lot and make it increasingly difficult to keep your arms by your sides.

Don't wear pants that are too baggy. You don't want your thumb or forefinger to get caught up in the baggy part of the crotch when you are performing swing type moves. Tight fitting shorts are a great idea.

Safety

- o Ensure that there is a clear space of one square meter (3.3 square feet) around you when you are working with kettlebells.
- o If you get in trouble with a rep, don't try to save the rep – simply move out of the way and let gravity take over.
- o If you can, use chalk to prevent your hands from becoming too slippery.
- o Have a towel on hand to wipe off sweat.
- o Stay hydrated throughout the workout.
- o Wear wristbands to prevent chaffing of the wrists and forearms.
- o Wear shoes with hard, flat soles.
- o Always lift and lower the kettlebell under control (bend you lower back!)

Kettlebell Movement Technique

Most kettlebell exercises will involve one of two grips:

- Finger hook grip
- Hand insertion grip

A palm up grip begins by inserting your middle finger through the middle of the kettlebell. Place the index finger under the thumb to create a finger grip hook.

You should avoid the following common grip mistakes:

- Gripping the handle too tight
- Holding the handle too loosely
- Holding only with the fingertips

Kettlebell Breathing Technique

There are two types of breathing used with kettlebell training; Paradoxical Breathing and Anatomical Breathing. When engaging in brief, heavy, high intensity training you should use paradoxical breathing. A set that lasts longer and uses a lighter weight should be accompanied by anatomical breathing.

Paradoxical Breathing

With this type of breathing you inhale during the eccentric part of the movement and exhale during the concentric part. As an example, with squats you would inhale on the way down and exhale on the way up.

Anatomical Breathing

Anatomical breathing is the reverse of paradoxical breathing – you inhale during the concentric part of the movement and exhale during the eccentric part. This type of breathing is ideal for endurance training.

II. The 13 Soviet Kettlebell Moves

Kettlebell Exercise No.1: Kettle Halo

The kettlebell halo, also known as "around the world", is an excellent exercise for core development, and shoulder strength. Grab the kettlebell from the outside of the horns, and bring it up to chin level, so that you are holding it upside down in a goblet squat position. The bottom of the kettlebell should be facing the ceiling. The elbows should be tucked in, in a rack position. Now drive the elbows to one side, so that the kettlebell goes over the shoulder and around to the back of the head. Be sure to keep your glutes clenched and your abs tight. Be sure, also, to keep your lower back flat. Bring the kettlebell over the other shoulder and back to the upside down goblet position at the front of your body.

Now change direction as you repeat the movement around the head and back to your chest. Your base position is both elbows tucked in at the chest. As you move you untuck one and then the other to facilitate the rotational movement. You should keep the path of the exercise comparable to a halo above the head. Try to keep the kettlebell close to the head throughout the movement. Don't allow your head to move throughout the exercise – keep it looking straight ahead. It helps to pick a spot on the wall in front of you and to keep your eyes focused on it throughout the movement. If you have to look down and drop the head then the kettlebell is too heavy. Lighten the load to allow proper technique.

Kettlebell Exercise No.2: Kettlebell Deadlift

The deadlift is a foundational exercise for developing strength in the posterior chain, including the muscles of the lower back, glutes and hamstrings. The kettlebell version also improves hip increasing technique, allowing for better performance on such exercises as snatches, cleans and swings.

Place the kettlebell on the floor between your legs and just in front of you. With your feet shoulder width apart, sit back with your hips, allowing yourself to go down until you can reach the handles. Keep your chest up throughout the movement. Now grab the handle with both hands and return to a standing position by pushing your heels into the ground. The power for the lift will come from your glutes, which should be squeezed tight, and your lower back (erector spine).

Next, repeat the descent by pushing the hips and gently lowering until the kettlebell just kisses the ground. It is important to keep the center of gravity aligned over your base while doing this movement. In addition, you should be creasing your body at the hips, rather than bending at the waist. Your lower back should be slightly arched throughout the movement. To target the hamstrings more, keep your legs straight throughout the movement. To place more emphasis on the glutes, bend your legs slightly on the descent. Keep your elbows back and chest up throughout the movement.

A variation on this movement is a double kettlebell deadlift, grabbing the kettlebells in a grocery bag type lift.

Kettlebell Exercise No.3: Two Handed Kettlebell Swing

The kettlebell swing is a classic kettlebell power developer. In order to perfect the technique follow a two-step process as outlined below:

Step One: With feet shoulder width apart, place the kettlebell between your toes. As in the deadlift, thrust you hips back to go down to the kettlebell (imagine that you are trying to close a car door with your butt). Keep your head up, ensuring that your shoulders don't get ahead of your knees. Grab the kettlebell with a two handed overhand grip. Rise up to a standing position quickly, popping your hips as you come up. Do this five times in rapid succession.

Step Two: Place the kettlebell back further so that the handle is in line with your heels. Repeat the movement that you have just performed. You will notice that, this time, there is a small pendulum effect at the top of the movement. Now try to drive the kettlebell back between your legs as you go down, so that it goes down, under your butt. On the ascent, pop the weight up to just below shoulder level. Be sure that you are not lifting with your arms or shoulders – the power must originate from the hips. This is one exercise where a pendulum like swing is desired. The use of momentum in this way reduces the strain on the lower back and grip while allowing for greater work capacity.

Kettlebell Exercise No.4: One Arm Clean

The one arm clean is a great intermediary movement between swing and pressing exercises. As you become proficient at this movement, you should develop a rhythmic motion, which flows from one rep into the next.

It's important that you maintain a loose grip on the kettlebell during this movement. This will prevent the bell from banging on your forearm as you perform the exercise. Begin with a slightly wider than shoulder width stance and the kettlebell sitting between your legs. Thrust your hips back, with lower back arched slightly, to come down and grip the kettlebell, with and over-hand grip, your thumb pointed behind you. Your non-working hand should be out to the side, with the fist closed. Maintain a good back posture with your head up.

Inhale as you clean the kettlebell to shoulder level. As you rise up, the kettlebell should swivel in your hand into a lock position. When you lock out at the top position, your glutes, quads and hamstrings should all be tight. As you rise, the kettlebell should move vertically up your body. At the top position, allow the kettlebell to rest on your chest and forearm in what is known as the rack position. The kettlebell should now be sitting in the triangle that is formed by the elbow, forearm and chest.

A common problem with this movement is uncomfortable banging of the kettlebell on the forearm. This occurs because you are gripping the handle too tight. Loosen the grip, allowing the fingers to go as deeply into the handle as possible as the kettlebell comes up to chest level.

Kettlebell Exercise No.5: Single Press

Begin with the kettlebell in the top position of the One Arm Clean (the rack position). Your elbow should be tucked into your stomach and your wrist and arm should be in a straight line. Put your non -working arm out to the side for stability. Drive the kettlebell up in a straight line until your elbow is completely locked out in the top position. Your hand should be positioned such that your thumb is pointing directly back behind you. Make sure that you are pushing with the whole body, as opposed to just the shoulders. The movement needs to include the flaring of the lats and the compression and extension of the spine.

Lower the kettlebell by moving your body slightly back to allow the kettlebell to return to the rack position. The up-down movement needs to be fluid, without any jerking movements.

Breathing should follow a four-stage pattern as follows:

(1) Breath in deeply while holding the kettlebell in the rack position
(2) Breath out just prior to the overhead push
(3) Inhale as you drive up
(4) Exhale as you lock out in the top position

Kettlebell Exercise No.6: Snatch

The kettlebell snatch is built off the kettlebell swing, so make sure that your form is on point for the swing before moving to this exercise. With feet shoulder width apart, place the kettlebell between your toes. Thrust you hips back to go down to the kettlebell. Keep your head up, ensuring that your shoulders don't get ahead of your knees. Grab the kettlebell with a one handed overhand grip. Rise up to a standing position quickly, popping your hips as you come up. Make sure to keep your shins vertical throughout the movement.

Get a good pendulum motion going with several swings, with the hips initiating the movement, and the arms simply doing the guiding. Everything should be locked out in the top position. After about five swings, take the kettlebell all the way up until it is locked out overhead. As you go up, the kettlebell will swivel over your hand until, in the lockout position, it is resting against the back of your lower arm. In the top position your palm should be open. Re-grip on the way down. If you are doing high reps, hold the top position for a second or two in order to catch your breath. Alternate arms after every five overhead snatches.

Kettlebell Exercise No.7: Goblet Squat

The Kettlebell Goblet Squat is a fantastic movement for opening up the hips, and building power in the lower body. With a slightly wider than shoulder width grip, grab the kettlebell by the horns and hold it at chest level. Keep your elbows in as you descend into a squat. Actively pull yourself down, with your glutes and hips going out and back. Don't go back too far, however, because you want to stay as upright as possible. Go straight down into a full squat. The elbows should come down and rest inside your knees and against your inner thighs in the bottom squat position. This will prevent your knees from collapsing in. The knees will come forward slightly, but should not go inwards. Thrust your chest out and look up from this position. They should, in fact, track your toes at all times. In this bottom position, shift the knees from side to side, using your elbows to pry your thighs apart. Push your tailbone down and your head up.

Now take a deep breath, exhale and drive straight back up to the starting position.

Kettlebell Exercise No.8 Windmill

The Windmill is a very effective movement for the hamstrings, glutes, lower back and shoulders. It also targets the core, while making your stronger and more stable in the overhead position. This movement is also a great way to enhance your overall flexibility.

Start in the rack position with your feet shoulder width apart. Power the kettlebell up to a locked out overhead position. Angle your feet at a forty-five degree angle to the arm which is holding the kettlebell. Shift about 95 percent of your weight to the inside leg that is bearing the weight. Now kick the kettlebell side hip out, while you lower to take your non-kettlebell arm down towards the toe on the same side. Keep the overhead arm locked out as you descend. Look up throughout the movement, using your leg as a guide to track your arm down towards the toe.

It is optional as to whether you lock out the front leg. However, the back leg must stay locked out through the entire movement. Do not shift the weight to the front leg during the downward part of the movement. Rather keep your weight on the rear leg by pushing the rear hip up and back. Your shoulder will rotate as you thrust out your hip and lower your upper body to the toe.

Kettlebell Exercise No.9: High Pull

The Kettlebell High Pull is a whole body movement that builds power and functional strength that will make you more explosive for such sports as sprinting, basketball, boxing and karate.

With feet shoulder width apart, place the kettlebell between your toes. Thrust you hips back to go down to the kettlebell. Keep your head up, ensuring that your shoulders don't get ahead of your knees. Grab the kettlebell with a two handed overhand grip at the top of the horns so that your thumbs are touching. Make sure that your shoulders are in front of the weight. Begin the pull by pushing down through your feet and driving your hips up and forward. Keep your arms extended through this first part of the pull. Use the force of the leg drive to extend your body upward. Lift the kettlebell to chest level. Let your momentum carry you up on to your toes, then squat down to the start position. In the top position, your elbows should be elevated above the weight.

Kettlebell Exercise No.10: Turkish Get Up

The Turkish Get Up is a phenomenal total body exercise. It is great for cardiovascular conditioning as well for building functional strength and power. Start by lying on the floor, on your back with your knees bent. The kettlebell should be on the floor to your right. Place your right hand fully into the kettlebell handle and pull the weight to your chest. Now, with both shoulder blades on the floor, raise your right arm straight up so that the kettlebell is directly above your chest. The right knee should be bent so that the right foot is flat on the floor. Your left arm should be flat on the floor at a forty five degree angle.

From the start position, rise up onto your left elbow, keeping the right arm locked. From there, come up further so that you are supporting your body with just your left hand and your right foot. Your left leg should be straight and a few inches off the floor. Now move your butt and left leg back behind you to rest your left knee on the ground. You can now rise up to the lunge position, with your left hand off the floor and the points of contact now being your right foot and left shin. The kettlebell is still locked overhead.

Pushing off the back leg rise to a standing position. Keep your focus up on the kettlebell the whole time. Now reverse the exact motion to return to the start position.

Kettlebell Exercise No.11: Russian Twist

The Russian Twist is a very good movement to develop phenomenal core strength, while shaping and defining the obliques. Sit upright on the floor with a kettlebell alongside you, then lean back a little so that your abs are tensed to keep you up. Bend your knees and, keeping your legs together; elevate the feet to about six inches off the floor. Grab hold of the kettlebell with an overhand grip towards the top of the horns. Starting with the kettlebell sitting at your waist, rotate to the right to bring the weight to the floor. Once it touches, immediately rotate to the other side and touch the floor there. Repeat back and forth, making sure that you touch the kettlebell to the floor each time. You need to also ensure that your feet are off the ground throughout the entire motion.

Kettlebell Exercise No.12: Two Arm Kettlebell Row

This is a great exercise for developing functional strength in the muscle of the upper back, arms and shoulders. Start by placing a pair of kettlebells on the floor wide enough apart that you can step through them. Keeping your heels on the floor, bend down to grab the kettlebell handles. Let your hips track back and maintain an arch in your lower back as you go down. From there, soften your knees and push your glutes into the air. This will ensure a flat back position. Now breathe in as you pull your arms up to your chest. Keep the tension in the back muscles and the muscles of the upper arm. Control the kettlebells as you return them to the start position. Don't let the shoulders roll forward.

Kettlebell Exercise No.13: Lunge Clean / Lunge Press

This is a fluid movement that allows you to get a great power / cardio combination workout. It is beneficial for your heart and lungs and is a tremendous fat burner. Start by holding a kettlebell at your right side, with feet shoulder width apart. Now lunge forward with your right leg. As you come out of the lunge, clean the kettlebell to your right shoulder. Now continue moving forward by lunging with your left foot. As you come out of this lunge, press the kettlebell overhead. Continue this lunge-clean-lunge-process for the required time allotment.

III. Optimized Soviet Kettlebell Routines

In this chapter, we'll present you with training regimens targeted toward 2 distinct training goals:

- o Fat Loss
- o Muscle Gain

We'll give you 3 workouts for each of these goals, allowing you to progress your training from beginner to advanced level.

The Tabata Protocol

Your Fat Loss workouts will incorporate an advanced cardio regimen that will ramp you fat burn into the stratosphere. It's called the Tabata Protocol

The Tabata Protocol all began with the Japanese Olympic Speed Skating Team. The Head Coach, Irisawa Koichi, created a High Intensity Interval Training Workout for his skaters. This consisted of 8 rounds. Each round was 20 seconds of intense work using a cycling ergometer followed by 10 seconds of rest. Koichi had one of his training coaches, Azumi Tabata, analyze the effectiveness of this workout using scientific methods. This is where the Tabata Protocol (which HIIT training is based upon) came about. Tabata didn't actually invent the training method, but because of widespread interest in his findings the workout was named after him. Tabata's studies showed his subjects producing impressive results that make traditional (steady state) cardio seem ineffective by comparison.

To perform the Tabata Protocol with Kettlebells simply perform the movement for 20 seconds and then take a 10 seconds rest. Repeat for the stated number of sets.

The Fat Loss Workouts

Beginner Workout for Fat Loss

Warm-Up

- *Around-the-body pass :* 30 s each direction with light kettlebell
- *Halo :* 30 s each direction with light kettlebell
- *Kettlebell deadlift:* 10 reps
- *Goblet squat :* 10 reps

Workout

- *Two Handed Kettlebell Swing:* Tabata protocol for 20 s with 10 s rest before alternating arms. Repeat for 4 sets with 1 min recovery between sets.
- *Single Press:* Tabata protocol for 20 s with 10 s rest before alternating arms. Repeat for 4 sets with 1 min recovery between sets.

Warm-Down

- *Easy jog for 10 min*
- *Stretch for 5 min*: 30 s each side for each stretch (behind-the-back shoulder stretch; shoulder stretch, triceps pulls, standing knee-to-chest stretch, standing quadriceps stretch

Intermediate Workout for Fat Loss

Warm-Up

- o *Two-arm single-leg kettlebell deadlift :* 8 reps on each side
- o *Windmill :* 10 reps on each side
- o *Joint mobility exercises :* Rotate all major joints (shoulders, hips, neck) 10-20 times.

Workout

Perform as many rounds as possible in 10 min:

- o *Double swing :* 15 reps with medium-weight kettlebells
- o *Double clean :* 15 reps with medium-weight kettlebells
- o *Double front squat :* 15 reps with medium-weight kettlebells
- o *Russian twist :* 40 twists with medium-weight kettlebell

Warm-Down

- o *Easy jog for 10 min*
- o *Stretch for 5 min*: 30 s each side for each stretch (behind-the-back shoulder stretch; shoulder stretch, triceps pulls, standing knee-to-chest stretch, pg. standing quadriceps stretch

Advanced Workout for Fat Loss

Warm-Up

- *Easy jog for 5 min*
- *Dynamic mobility exercises:* arm twirls forward and backward for 30s, dynamic   clapping for 30 s, leg swings in each direction for 30 s

Workout

- *Goblet squat :* 30 s each side
- *Spinal flexion :* hold for 1 min
- *Calf stretch :* 1 min per leg

- *Two Arm Kettlebell Row:* Tabata protocol for 20 s with 10 s rest. Repeat for 4 sets.
- *Lunge Clean / Lunge Press:* Tabata protocol for 20 s with 10 s rest. Repeat for 4 sets.
- *Static stretches*: 30 s each side or 10 reps each exercise (standing quadriceps stretch; standing hamstrings stretch; standing knee-to-chest stretch; calf stretch; spinal flexion)

The Muscle Gain Workouts

Beginner Workout for Muscle Gain

- *Easy jog for 5 min*
- *Joint mobility exercises:* Rotate all major joints (shoulders, hips, neck) 10-20 times or for 5 min.
- Perform 10 reps of each of the following exercises on each side of the body without stopping. Repeat for 3 rounds with 1 min rest between each round. One round consists of the single swing, single clean, single press, snatch, and goblet squat.
- *Stretch for 7 min*: Perform each stretch for 1 min (behind-the-back shoulder stretch; standing knee-to-chest stretch; standing hamstrings stretch; standing quadriceps stretch; spinal extension; child's pose; spinal flexion).

Intermediate Workout for Muscle Gain

Warm-Up

- o *Easy jog for 5 min*
- o *Body-weight squat:* 1 set for 30 s
- o *Joint mobility exercises:* 20 reps of each (hip circles, trunk twists, lateral bends, waist bends, shoulder rolls, neck tilts, neck rotations, ankle bounces).

Workout

- o *Rack hold:* Hold for 2 min with two light kettlebells, rest 1 min, hold 2 min with two moderate-weight kettlebells, rest 2 min, hold 1 min with two heavy kettlebells.
- o *Overhead hold:* Hold 1 min with two light kettlebells, rest 1 min, hold 1 min with two moderate-weight kettlebells.
- o *Single Arm Press:* Do 2 sets of 5 reps per hand, resting 1 min between sets.
- o *Two Arm Kettlebell Rows:* Do 3 sets of 10 reps, resting 1 min between sets.
- o *Russian Twist:* Do 3 sets of 15 reps, resting 1 min between each set.
- o *Farmer's Carry:* Hold two heavy kettlebells for as long as possible for 1 set.

Warm-Down

- o *Easy jog for 5 min*
- o *Stretch for 7 min*: Perform each stretch for 1 min (behind-the-back shoulder stretch; standing knee-to-chest stretch; standing hamstrings stretch; standing quadriceps stretch; spinal extension; child's pose; spinal flexion).

Advanced Workout for Muscle Gain

Warm-Up

- *Body-weight squat:* 1 set of 30 reps
- *Skipping rope:* 1 min
- *Dynamic mobility exercises:* 15 reps of each arm twirls in both directions; chest hollow and expand; vertical chest opener; dynamic clapping; leg swings

Workout

- *Turkish Get-up:* 5 reps each arm
- *Goblet Squat:* 5 sets of 5 reps, resting 1 min between sets
- *One Arm Clean:* 1 min, rest 1 min
- *Snatch:* 1 min, rest 1 min
- *High Pull:* 5 sets of 10 reps, resting 1 min between sets

Warm-Down

- *Easy jog for 10 min*
- *Stretch for 7 min*: Perform each stretch for 1 min (behind-the-back shoulder stretch; standing knee-to-chest stretch; standing hamstrings stretch; standing quadriceps stretch; spinal extension; child's pose; spinal flexion).

IV. Final Word

By now you have developed a whole new respect for that daunting looking rack of bowling balls with handles that proliferate the gym floor. You've discovered that kettlebells are the key to unlocking your fat burn, allowing you to develop functional fitness and packing quality muscle onto your frame.

We encourage you to continue your kettlebell journey as you move progressively to the realization of your ideal body. Keep pushing, continue setting new goals and strive to be the best you can be.

Now that you've got the kettlebell advantage, never relinquish it!

Sage Surefire

Subscribe to our list to get notified of new book releases from Sage Surefire. We notify you of new book releases, updates to the books, and when a book is given away free.

http://eepurl.com/bronjj

You'll like my other books.

Women Bodybuilding: Build a lean, sexy, toned, curvy body without getting bulky

http://www.amazon.com/gp/product/B00YB9SAN0?*Version*=1&*entries*=0

CrossFit Training: Build a lean, athletic, sexy body with fresh and exciting crossfit workouts

http://www.amazon.com/gp/product/B00Z14BENW?*Version*=1&*entries*=0

Building Muscle: Bullshit free secrets to building muscle

http://www.amazon.com/gp/product/B010INJBPS?*Version*=1&*entries*=0

HIIT Workouts: Get HIIT fit, fast-track your way to a shredded, super-fit new you

http://www.amazon.com/gp/product/B010MSYK96?*Version*=1&*entries*=0